Multiple Sclerosis Tamed

By Lynne D M Noble

This book shall not, by way of trade or otherwise, be lent, re-sold, hired out, or otherwise circulated without the prior consent of the copyright holder or the publisher in any form of binding or cover than that in which it is published and without a similar condition including this condition being imposed on the subsequent purchaser. The use of its contents in another media is also subject to the same conditions.

Copyright 2019 Lynne D M Noble

Independently published

Contents

Preface………….. page iv

Vitamin D – the immune system modulator –page 1

Taurine: wonder molecule…. page 27

Effects of sodium on the progression of MS ……. page 30

Comparison of amino acids in the serum of meat and fish eating individuals … page 33

Fish and alanine ……. page 38

Building blocks of myelin sheath …… page 42

Vitamin C and re-myelination …. page 45

Vitamin B complex ….. page 49

MS and the virus connection …… page 60

Thiamine…… page 63

Thiamine sources, functions and other miscellany…… page   77

Vitamin C deficiency and MS ….. page 85

Putting it all together ……. Page 93

Dedication

To Greta Reid

with every blessing

About the Author

Lynne Noble was born in 1953 in Huddersfield, West Yorkshire. From a very early age, Lynne showed an interest in nutrition and genetics avidly reading any books that she could get her hands on at the time.

Initially, Lynne studied orthopaedics but events led her to work with the elderly mentally infirm. Here, her interest in neurodegenerative disorders and pain syndromes developed.

Lynne undertook rigorous programmes of study, completing her Cert Ed., (FE) BSc (Hons) and Adv. Dip Education simultaneously before moving onto her M.Ed.

From there she took further demanding programmes in Human Nutrition, Pharmacology, Neuroscience, Genetics and Immunology. During this time, she was given many prestigious awards for her academic work. It was noted then that Lynne was not afraid of tackling difficult subjects.

She began her law degree but ill health prevented her from pursuing this. However, in this time, she moved from being a foster parent to adoptive parent.

She has been instrumental in setting up projects in the community for disadvantaged groups.

She is a member of the Guild of Health Writers.

Now retired, she lives with her husband in a historic Georgian riverside town in the West Midlands. She enjoys gardening, watching her husband bowling and researching.

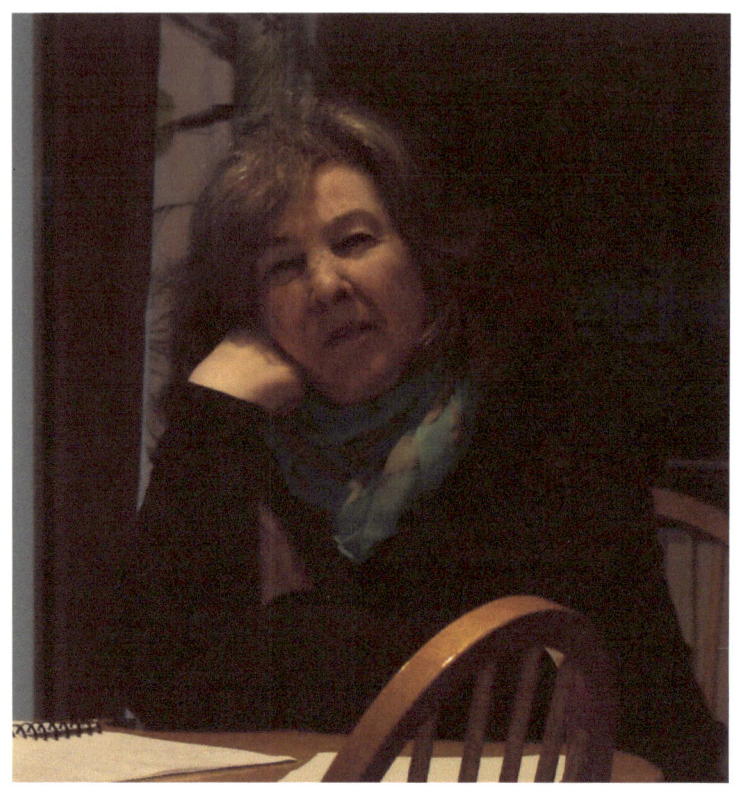

Author Lynne Noble at home

https://quintessentiallylynne.weebly.com/nutritional-medicine.html

Preface

Multiple Sclerosis is a complex condition which affects over 2.3 million people worldwide. In reality this figure will be even higher since many people with troubling symptoms will not have yet been referred to a consultant for diagnosis.

[1]The National MS Society describes the condition thus:

Multiple Sclerosis is a chronic, unpredictable disease of the central nervous system (CNS), which is made up the brain, spinal cord and optic nerves. It is thought to be an immune mediated disorder, in which the immune system incorrectly attacks healthy tissue in the CNS.

MS can be classified by type. There are:

- Clinically isolated. That is, a first episode of neurological symptoms caused by

---

[1] https://www.nationalmssociety.org/

inflammation and demyelination in the central nervous system.
- Relapsing and remitting MS where there are periods of relapses. Following relapses, there is partial or full recovery.
- Primary progressive MS follows a general decline in disability over a long period. There may be relapses but these are few and far between.
- Secondary progressive MS follows the pattern of the relapsing-remitting type and develops into a more general decline with or without relapses.

Most of the initial symptoms of this condition are not recognised as symptomatic of MS. They may include:

- Areas of numbness or pins and needles
- Eye pain – often misdiagnosed as migraine
- Tripping up – often misdiagnosed as 'having a clumsy day.'

The symptoms occur when there is inflammation, produced by immune system, that attacks the myelin sheath.

This is a type of insulation which protects the nerve.

The inflammation also damages a type of cell known as an 'oligodendrocyte' which makes the myelin in the central nervous system.

Sometimes, the damage can actually extend to the nerve fibre.

An oligodendrocyte is a cell, found in the central nervous system, that secretes myelin sheath around the nerve.

It plays a similar role to the Schwann cell, that is found in the peripheral nervous system and which wraps their cell body around the axon as myelination occurs.

Treatment has moved on considerably in the last few years for those who have MS. There are many disease modifying drugs but they do not come without side effects.

Nevertheless, disease modifying drugs do not stop the disease from manifesting itself in the first place, nor do they help the patient address this condition through other means.

MS prevalence has increased by 6.7 times since 1961 and between 1996 and 2011, the incidence of the disease has increased by more than two and a half times.[2] Women are most affected.

The Swank diet which was popularised in the 1950's has not lived up to expectations. It proposed a very low fat diet.

This was based on Swank's knowledge that people living on the coast who mainly had a fish diet were less likely to get MS than those who lived in the mountains and whose main form of protein was meat and egg.

Swank proposed that those with MS should limit their diets to

---

[2] https://www.smh.com.au/lifestyle/why-more-women-than-ever-are-being-diagnosed-with-ms-20171023-gz68q8.html

- no more than 15gms of saturated fat daily and
- no more than 50g of total fat per day
- 20g -35g of unsaturated fat per day

The unsaturated oils that Swank proposed were beneficial have now been found to cause inflammation.

In MS, we are trying to reduce inflammation, not increase it!

Some fats which Swank did not recommend would actually be healthy in that they contain good amounts of vitamin D. As we shall see, vitamin D is vital in the health of the central nervous system.

A very low fat diet, such as Swank's is not healthy given that there are four fat soluble vitamins which are absolutely essential to neurological health and need fat to be absorbed.

For those following the Swank diet it was recommended that supplements containing certain vitamin and minerals be taken.

This does not make sense to withdraw them from the diet and then replace them through supplements.

Swank's diet was found to cause extremely dry skin and hair.

Swank's research did not have a control group and there was a high drop-out rate. The latter is not surprising since a low fat diet is generally unpalatable.

A further diet called the McDougall diet was studied in 2016. This was an onerous diet – and again very low fat. However, it also excluded all meat, fish, eggs, dairy and vegetable oils.

The results of those individuals who participated showed that their brain scans did not indicate improvement or fewer relapses.

Their BMI's however, did change. It was referred to as a positive change in that the participants lost weight. However, weight loss is not always to be sought as it can be the result of the loss of muscle mass and not fat.

We need to retain as much muscle mass as possible - not lose it - through unwise eating.

Cholesterol and insulin levels were lower in the diet group after six months, than when the participants first started, but they were higher when the study ended.

Therefore, it does not appear that there is a positive correlation between the amount of fat eaten and cholesterol levels.

The liver makes cholesterol which is an essential substance in the body.

25% of the total cholesterol, that is synthesised, is found in the brain.

High levels of cholesterol, in recent studies,[3] have been found to ward against infections.

Cholesterol has antioxidant and anti-inflammatory effects. As such cholesterol would have beneficial effects on the health of the brain.

---

[3] https://www.medicalnewstoday.com/articles/318598.php?sr

Clearly, there were other unknown factors at work which might account for the differences in the incidences of MS between Swank's populations but it was not as a result of saturated fat differences.

There are clear differences in the nutrients found in a mainly fish diet when contrasted with the predominantly meat and egg diet which formed the diet of the mountain dwelling people. When we examine these differences in more detail, they form the basis of a healthy bespoke diet for those who have been diagnosed with MS.

We know that chronic inflammation 'nibbles' away at the myelin sheath which is produced by myelin producing cells called oligodendrocytes.

It is therefore in our interest to not only regulate these inflammatory processes but respond to any chronic inflammation since it serves no useful purpose. Fortunately, this is not an onerous task.

My intentions in writing this book are:

1. To inform. This will include understanding of what a bespoke diet for MS, which promotes brain health and reduces inflammation, consists of.

2. To present this material in an easily read and easily understood form, bearing in mind that this book is for those with multiple sclerosis and their families. As such, I will not be including any 'heavy' research in the book although the information in this book is research based. Such a book may well come later but it is not for now

3 To learn a little about the antioxidants which promote good brain health and which help to prevent further neurodegeneration.

4 to examine the differences between the diets of the coastal inhabitants and mountain dwellers and how these differences in the nutritional composition can support neurological health.

5 to examine other nutritional substances which positively impact the health of the brain and myelin sheath.

Please note, I am not proposing a diet which is primarily a fish one. This would be unacceptable to many as fish is not to everyone's taste.

There is no doubt that diet does make a difference to the progression of multiple sclerosis and our understanding of this is increasing all the time.

It is about time that we begin to look at nutrition and how it impacts MS.

Vitamin D – the Immune System 'Regulator' which is necessary for brain health

Vitamin D is essential for the overall health of the body including the brain.

It is a fat soluble vitamin and cannot be absorbed without the presence of some fat in the diet. Therefore, low fat or no fat diets may aid the progression of multiple sclerosis. Further, vitamin D needs to be activated and it cannot do this without the presence of sufficient magnesium. Both magnesium and vitamin D are known to be generally insufficient in about 80% of people.

Not one nutrient acts in isolation which is why a diverse diet is always recommended.

Receptors for vitamin D are found in every organ and tissue of the body and this gives us an indication of how important this vitamin is

Vitamin D receptors are tiny shapes on cells. They grab onto vitamin D. More receptors are expressed on the surface of a cell if there is greater need for it at any particular time.

Receptors would not be found on cells if that cell did not need vitamin D to fulfil its function.

Cells that receive vitamin D, can be found throughout the body and there is marked intracellular distribution of vitamin D receptors in the brain.

Developmental vitamin D deficiency has been found to cause abnormal brain development.

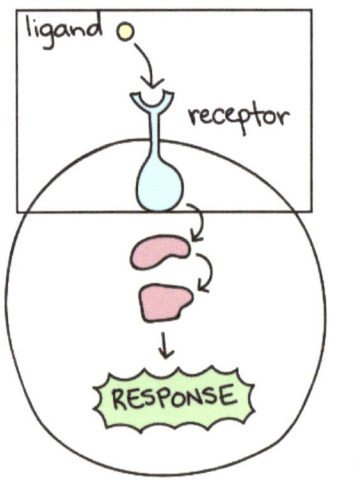

---

[4] https://www.khanacademy.org/science/biology/cell-signaling/mechanisms-of-cell-signaling/a/signal-perception

Studies[5] have shown an association between low vitamin D levels with a greater amount of relapses and lesions in patients with MS. Further other studies have shown that when 10,000 international units of this vitamin was taken every day for six months, it reduced the number of specific immune cells that are known to cause damage in MS.

There was a slower decline in progression scores when patients were treated with 2000 IU's of cholecalciferol daily compared to the control group who did not receive any vitamin D.

Most people are aware that vitamin D is necessary to build strong bones but it has many other important roles to play in health including a regulatory role in the immune system.

This regulatory role – important in auto immune conditions – also inhibits rampant microglia which play such an important part in the progression of multiple sclerosis.

---

[5] https://www.mssociety.org.uk/research/explore-our-research/emerging-research-and-treatments/vitamin-d

Microglia are a specific population of immune cells that are found in the central nervous system. Their function is to removed damaged neurons (brain cells) and infections.

They are vitally important for maintaining the health of the brain.

In MS patients, destruction of myelin in the CNS is associated with activated macrophages or microglia.

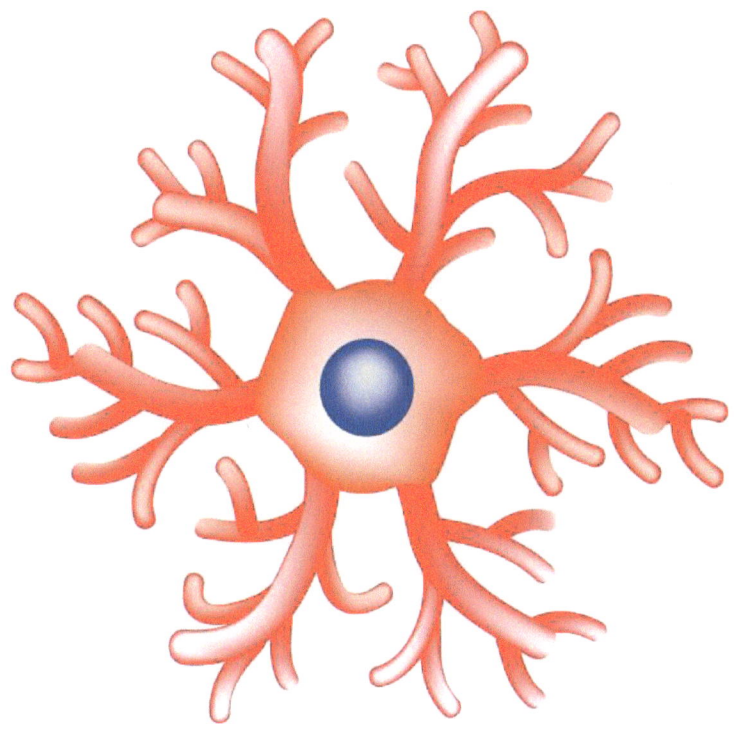

An activated microglial cell grows lots of arms.

These microglia above have become activated because they have come into contact with damaged or infected cells. Non activated microglia do not have the protrusions on their cell body.

Sometimes microglia can't differentiate between healthy brain tissue and infected tissue. They begin to attack healthy brain tissue in MS.

This is what causes chronic inflammation that is characteristic of the progression of MS.

Sufficient vitamin D – either in diet, sun exposure or supplements - can stop this from occurring. This Is because vitamin D activates the innate and the acquired immune system when infection strikes so that the immune system can deal with the infective agent.

Although vitamin D is an important vitamin in slowing or stopping the progression of MS, it is practically impossible to get enough from the diet. There are very few foods that contain it and many of these foods do not form a regular part of many people's diet.

Further, as we grow older we become less efficient at absorbing most nutrients in our diet and, as appetite lessens with age, we take in fewer nutrients. These factors all contribute to vitamin D deficiency.

Vitamin D requires fat to aid its absorption, yet our current propensity to very low fat – or no fat - diets hinders this.

Fortunately, this vitamin is also made through the action of sunlight on the skin. The easiest way to get Vitamin D is to expose your skin to sunlight. However, the amount of vitamin D which can be made in this way depends on:

- the colour of your skin,
- how much skin is exposed and
- the intensity of the sun's ultraviolet B rays.
- It is also dependent on the amount of cholesterol you have in your body, since it is the action of the sun's rays on the cholesterol under the skin which helps synthesise vitamin D.

Therefore, the action of some medications which reduce the synthesis of cholesterol could be a risk factor for multiple sclerosis.

The current fashion of covering up and slapping sun cream on as soon as the sun appears could be causing more harm than good in many respects. I can understand that our pale skins would need some protection if exposed to prolonged intense sunshine such as that found in some countries where the sun's rays are much stronger than to be found in ours. However, most of the time we live in an environment where the sun's rays are quite weak and we should not inhibit our capacity to make vitamin D.

Most people understand that vitamin D is necessary for strong healthy bones but they may not be aware that vitamin D synthesises an antimicrobial peptide called cathelicidin which helps us fight infection.

It is not well known that vitamin D has an essential regulatory function, in the brain and body, by helping to prevent auto immunity. We shall look at autoimmunity in some detail later because it may not be all that it is considered to be.

Cathelicidin is important; it is one of the innate immune system's range of defences. Cathelicidin related antimicrobial peptides (CAMP) are key compounds of the innate immune system.

The innate immune system is the general defence system which you are born with. It does not consist of antibodies which are part of the more specialised acquired immune system.

The general (innate) immune system consists of the skin and mucous membranes, temperature, neutrophils, monocytes and Natural Killer Cells, among others.

General immune system cells have a broad spectrum anti-microbial action again gram+ and gram - bacteria, viruses and fungi.

They have immune modulatory functions including roles in wound healing, the induction of cytokines and altering gene expression.[6]

---

[6] https://www.ncbi.nlm.nih.gov/pubmed/280821

Cathelicidin is important because a bacterium *Clostridium perfringens* was found to be elevated in those with MS. This bacterium produces an epsilon toxin which is able to disrupt the blood brain barrier and cross it.

In animals it produces devastating disease.

This bacterium is found in the soil and flourishes in poorly cooked meat. This could explain the difference which Swank noticed in the diet of his study groups where the meat and egg eaters, were significantly more likely to have MS, than fish eaters.

Nevertheless, studies have shown that sufficient vitamin D can address any adverse effects from the epsilon toxin.

Studies have also shown that when there was a deficiency of the anti-microbial peptide, cathelicidin, it was associated with a more marked pro-inflammatory response.

CAMP deficient mice displayed a higher degree of microglial cell activation that was accompanied by a more pronounced pro-inflammatory response.

Exposure to the sun for thirty minutes, at least twice a week, should produce adequate amounts of vitamin D for our needs in the summer. However, getting enough vitamin D naturally, through the winter time, is far more problematical. It is at this time that supplementation with this vitamin needs to be considered for optimum health.

The Recommended Dietary Allowance (RDA) for Vitamin D was originally set at 400 International Units (IU's) in the 1950's.

This decision was based on the minimum amount required to prevent rickets – that was all. This amount cannot adequately sustain a healthy body nor maintain optimum neurological health.

There is a huge difference between 'just preventing' illness and 'optimising' overall health.

The current recommendation for vitamin D are between 1,000 and 4,000 IU's daily especially in the winter months when the levels of sunlight are not adequate.

The best form to take is Vitamin D3 which is the active form. Vitamin D is also available as vitamin D2 but this needs to go through an extra metabolic step to change it into the active part.

Many supplements come as dry powders, in capsule form or tablets. If these are swallowed by themselves without fat, then they will be of little use in raising vitamin D levels. Vitamin D does need to be taken with some fat.

Blood tests can easily identify whether you have too little or too much of this vitamin so anyone who has a neurodegenerative disorder should ask for a blood test, from their GP, to establish vitamin D levels. However, caution here; the levels of vitamin D that the medical establishment tends to think is adequate is generally well below of that needed to begin to turn around multiple sclerosis.

The National Institute of Health has provided these serum concentrations as a guide.[7]

Table 1: Serum 25-Hydroxyvitamin D [25(OH)D] Concentrations and Health [1]

nmol/L*	ng/mL*	Health status
<30	<12	Associated with vitamin D deficiency, which can lead to rickets in infants and children and osteomalacia in adults
30 to <50	12 to <20	Generally considered inadequate for bone and overall health in healthy individuals
≥50	≥20	Generally considered adequate for bone and overall health in healthy individuals
>125	>50	Linked to potential adverse effects,

[7] https://ods.od.nih.gov/factsheets/VitaminD-HealthProfessional/

Table 1: Serum 25-Hydroxyvitamin D [25(OH)D] Concentrations and Health [1]

nmol/L*	ng/mL*	Health status
		particularly at >150 nmol/L (>60 ng/mL)

Although the recommendation is not to ascertain levels of vitamin D in healthy people, it seems to me that this would be a judicious move if this was undertaken in September prior to the seasonal respiratory infection season and any insufficiency corrected before winter. This would reduce the overall burden that winter brings to the local GP practice and the hospitals considerably.

It probably comes as no surprise that MS sufferers tend to have more than their fair share of respiratory infections since there is an underlying common cause.

Vitamin D deficiency is associated with weak regulation of the immune response.

Studies[8] have found quantitatively, that lower than optimum levels of concentration of active vitamin D corresponded to weak regulation of the immune response. This means that once a pathogen/antigen enters the body, the nature of the immune response would be less regulatory, and hence more aggressive or inflammatory.

The immune system will respond to any infective agent by producing effector T-cells. These are involved in the autoimmune response.

A deficiency of vitamin D = out of control inflammation

---

[8] https://arxiv.org/abs/1304.7193

> *Low vitamin D levels = less regulation of effector T cells.*
>
> *The effector T cells will go into overdrive and attack your own tissue.*
>
> *This will result in further inflammation'*

Effector T cells are involved in the body's defences. Generally, many more effector T cells than are needed, are produced.

Unfortunately, these effector T cells don't always distinguish between what is foreign material and what isn't. As such, effector T cells may start destroying their own host's tissues.

If this scenario occurs in the brain, chronic neuro-inflammation and neurodegeneration may occur.

Optimum vitamin D levels reduce this hyperactivity which is characteristic of unregulated effector T cells.

Vitamin D can be synthesised from the action of sunlight on the cholesterol which is found just below the skin's surface. Insufficient cholesterol will jeopardise the synthesis of vitamin D.

Vitamin D helps regulate microglia so that they don't attack 'self' tissue so it is vitally important that we have sufficient levels, however this is obtained.

Those people who are particularly likely to be at risk of a vitamin D deficiency.

- Older People – because

Skin gets thinner as you get older. This makes it harder to make Vitamin D when it is exposed to sunlight.

Older people tend to eat less and also tend to spend more time indoors – both these will reduce the amount of vitamin D someone has in their system.

- People with Darker Skin because

The melanin in their skin helps protect them from the sun's ultra violet rays which reduces the body's ability to make this vitamin from the sun.

- People with medical conditions which reduce fat absorption and those on low fat diets because

Vitamin D is fat soluble and needs a properly functioning gut to be able to absorb fat from the diet. As vitamin D is fat soluble it cannot be found in foods which don't contain fat.

People who may be affected include those with Crohn's disease and liver disease due to fat absorption problems.

- Those who live further away from the equator or work indoors because

They are exposed to less sunlight.

- Those on cholesterol lowering drugs such as statins because

Cholesterol is required to make vitamin D

Dietary sources of Vitamin D

Cod Liver Oil: one tablespoon contains approximately 1,400 international units.

In the shorter months - from October until March - I would recommend two tablespoons daily for anyone with a neurodegenerative disease, or who belong to the susceptible groups already mentioned above.

- Cooked salmon: three ounces contains about 450 international units
- Beef liver: three ounces contains about 40 international units
- Egg yolk: one large, 40 international units
- irradiated mushrooms: three ounces, 35 international units.

As you can appreciate, it is difficult, if not impossible to take in up to 3000 IU's of vitamin D, daily.

It would be too simplistic to say that all manifestations of multiple sclerosis are simply due to insufficient vitamin D or magnesium or fat for absorption. The body is a hugely complex piece of machinery which is linked to many pathways. Disruption of any one of these can, and does, impact many other pathways. Think of a small cog in a huge piece of machinery and how this one small cog – or indeed any other part of the machinery anywhere - cause the whole of it to come to a standstill.

Thus we need to look further at this strange condition known as MS which may manifest itself as a relapsing remitting condition or as a progressive condition. Does it have multiple causes? Is it really a result of this autoimmunity going on or is it just a horrible manifestation of a simple nutritional deficiency?

The answer may surprise you in the end. There are many conditions which have devastating impacts on the lives of people which are just the result of a nutritional deficiency.

Very few nutritional deficiencies are ever tested for. Many are more expensive to carry out and so the cost implications forbid it being part of the GP's limited response to a patient complaint.

Further, GP's simply are taught very little about the impact of nutrients on the health of people. They are taught to respond to illness with a range of pharmaceutical products. That's their role.

Vitamins and minerals are very cheap and do not generate profits and we live in a largely profit driven world.

Granny's tried and tested remedies have largely been forgotten although they are slowly beginning to creep back.

In the 1950's, children were given cod liver oil, rose hip syrup and malt in order to increase the amount of vitamin A, D C and B vitamins that were generally in short supply immediately post war.

Now we have more and more foods where nutrients have been taken out and then substituted for similar, only the 'similar' may not be as bio available as the original.

Life styles change. The world has become more stressful and thus we need a greater intake of some vitamins like the B complex and vitamin C which are used up rapidly at the times of stress.

Adaptation is key.

The difference between the omega 3 fats in fish based and meat diets.

When I have asked people what foods they believe contain omega 3 fats, they are quick to point out that fish contains omega 3. When I ask about meat, they are not sure; most people say that it doesn't.

Surprisingly, both meat and fish contain sources of omega 3 but the types found in meat and fish are not the same.

In grass-fed beef there is something called alpha-linoleic acid (ALA) whereas the types found in fish are EPA (Eicosapentoaenoic acid) and DHA. (docosahexaenoic acid).

Some ALA can be converted to EPA and DHA but it is only tiny amounts; certainly not enough for optimum health.

Normally, ALA's benefits can be seen in relation to obesity, diabetes, cancer and heart disease but it is not generally associated with any major anti-inflammatory effects on the brain or, indeed, anywhere else in the body. As we are seeking to reduce inflammatory processes in the brain, then ALA is not something that we are likely to consider as being of as much use as other types of omega 3 such as EPA and DHA.

When we look at EPA and DHA, we find that their properties are different even though they are both a type of omega 3.

Firstly, DHA is a building block of tissue in the brain and retina of the eye. It, like EPA, has been found to be more biologically potent than ALA.

EPA and DHA have been found to have marked anti-inflammatory properties and therefore have great potential in ameliorating the inflammation that is fanning the progression of conditions like MS.

Studies[9] have shown that in placebo-controlled trials of fish oil, used in chronic inflammatory disease, there was significant benefit.

This would not be true of the ALA omega 3 which is a meat based fatty acid.

These differences in the meat and fish based omega three fatty acids could offer an explanation why a fish based diet is so beneficial for individuals with MS.

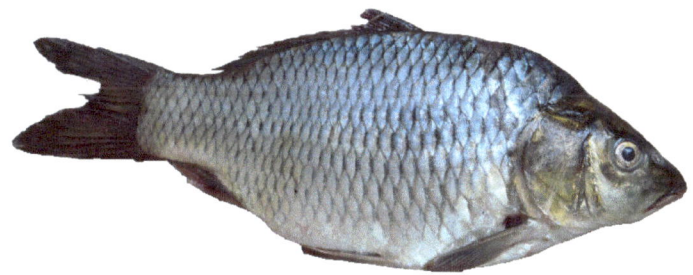

---

[9] https://www.ncbi.nlm.nih.gov/pubmed/12480795

In a nutshell, a fish based diet contains the anti-inflammatory fats DHA and EPA. Further, fish are not contaminated with *Clostridium Perfringens* which is associated with poorly cooked meat, nor is it contaminated with soil which is a rich source of this MS associated bacterium.

However, this isn't the only major difference in the nutritional status of a meat or fish based diet which may impact the progression of MS.

Diverse protein sources will be composed of different mixes of amino acids. Amino acids form cells and tissues and enzymes and without them we could not grow or repair injury or carry out life sustaining processes in the body.

One of these amino acids is mainly found in fish protein and only in limited amounts in other sources of animal protein.

It is an intriguing amino acid which is often mentioned on tins of cat food as it is essential for the health of cat's eyes.

We don't often associate it with longevity in humans.

We can now turn our attention to an amazing amino acid known as taurine.

Taurine: a wonder molecule

Taurine is a non-essential amino sulfonic acid which is found in large amounts in the brain, retina, platelets and heart.

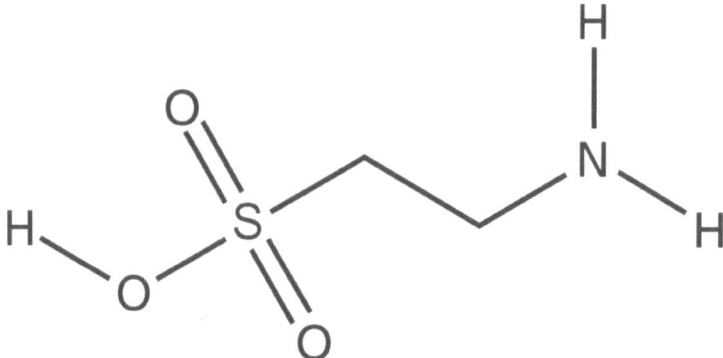

Taurine is a wonder molecule

It is not a constituent of a protein but it is found in the intracellular fluid of cells mainly belonging to the brain and heart. It can be synthesised from two other amino acids – cysteine and methionine but only in the presence of vitamin B_6.

Vitamin B_6 is a cofactor. This means that it is a non-protein 'helper' molecule that aids processes in the body.

The best sources of taurine are to be found in seafood especially mussels, scallops and clams. These are often eaten raw and, as such, retain far greater amounts of taurine. Taurine leaches into the cooking fluid which is then thrown away.

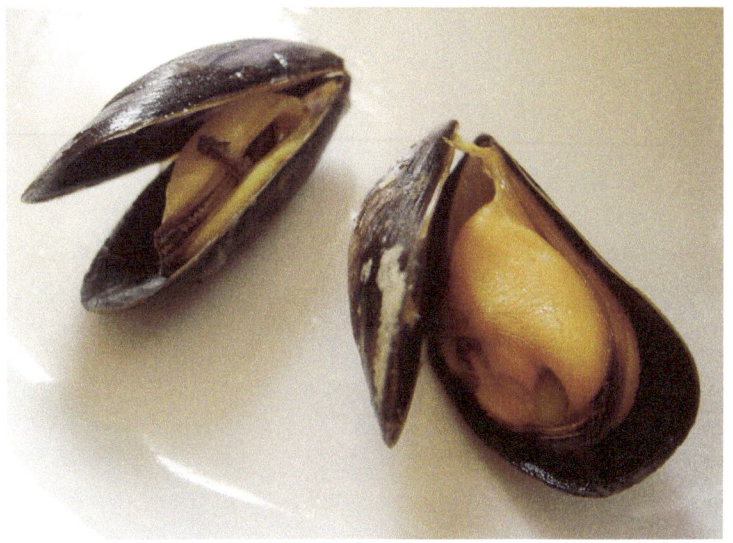

Mussels are a good source of tauring

Cooked meat contains only about 10mg of taurine per ounce whereas the same amount of a fish based product would yield four times as much.

The current recommended dosage of taurine is 500 – 2,000mg daily. Based on these amounts it is practically impossible to take in sufficient taurine through a meat and egg diet.

The people of Okinawa, where living to a hundred occurs here more than anywhere else in the world, have a largely fish based diet with lots of fresh vegetables.

Their longevity is attributed to their high taurine diet.

Taurine aids the cleansing of free radical waste and helps control many aspects of the ageing process.

It also helps provide neurotransmitter activity for many areas of the brain.

There is yet another benefit of taurine which also has important implications for people who have MS.

We shall turn to this in our next chapter.

The effects of a high salt diet on the progression of MS

There are now numerous studies which link multiple sclerosis with a high salt diet. Sodium is implicated in triggering the disease as well as exacerbation and progression of the disease.

A study[10] showed high salt diets disrupt T cells and cause increased inflammation. This is something we should be trying to avoid at all costs.

Although we do excrete excess salt, it is thought that some may remain in micro-domains – small regions in the cell membrane.

In addition, there are genetic differences in the way that excess sodium is dealt with in the body.

Some individuals appear to excrete excess sodium quite quickly but others may retain fluid and feel bloated.

More and more research has been undertaken on the impact of sodium after the initial study. The findings have been along similar lines.

This is when taurine comes into its own.

---

[10] https://www.nature.com/articles/s41590-018-0236-6

Taurine acts as a natural diuretic keeping magnesium and potassium in the cells and sodium out of them.

This also includes any sodium in the micro-domains which could cause inflammation in the brain.

Comparison of amino acids in serum of meat eating and fish eating individuals

A study[11] investigated the plasma concentrations and intakes of amino acids in male meat-eaters, fish eaters as well as vegetarians and vegans. For the purpose of this chapter I will examine the meat and fish based plasma concentrations.

There was little difference between the essential amino acids which are those that the individual has to get through diet since they cannot synthesise them within the body. However, there were some significant

---

[11] https://www.ncbi.nlm.nih.gov/pmc/articles/PMC4705437/

differences in the composition of the non-essential amino acids of those eating a meat based diet compared to those on mainly a fish based diet.

The one that we are concerned with is glutamate. Glutamate has major connections and functions in the brain.

It is a chemical messenger which is involved in neurodevelopment and neuro-proliferation under normal circumstances.

However, studies have shown that excessive activation of the glutamate receptors can lead to death of brain cells.

Studies have shown that excessive glutamate may be implicated in a number of diseases of the brain including MS.

Normal Glutamate = neuro-proliferation and neurodevelopment

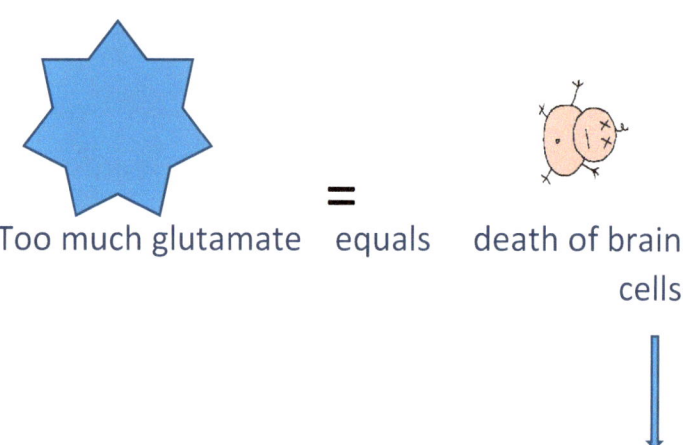

Too much glutamate equals death of brain cells

Death of brain cells will release greater amounts of ammonia which is neurotoxic

We should not be too alarmed about this though because studies show that sufficient amounts of vitamin D increase a substance called glutathione which is neuroprotective substance.

> Vitamin D produces glutathione which is neuroprotective.

Glutathione is an antioxidant produced in cells and it is composed of three amino acids:

- glutamine
- glycine
- cysteine

Glutathione levels are easily depleted through poor nutrition, stress and environmental toxins.

Ageing also reduces the amount of glutathione available in the body.

Now, even though (oily) fish contains more glutamate than meat, it also contains vitamin D which meat lacks. This means that fish is able to synthesise glutathione which is neuroprotective and can protect against an excess of glutamate. It is an in built protective device.

Normally excess glutamate is turned into a calming brain messenger known as GABA. However, autoimmune diseases and genetics can prevent this conversion from amino acid into a useful neurotransmitter.

Vitamin D protects us from this.

Ammonia is highly toxic to brain cells

Special brain cells called astrocytes protect against neurotoxicity by taking up excess glutamate and ammonia. Ammonia is highly toxic to brain cells.

Astrocytes convert these toxic substances into

> Astrocytes take up ammonia + glutamate and convert them to harmless glutamine

harmless glutamine.

Astrocytes can be overwhelmed if there is excessive ammonia. Too much ammonia causes the astrocytes to swell so they can't do their job properly.

Ammonia is produced when protein is broken down. This can happen during damage to cells through injury or infection.

And it is the ammonia made in the body, and not just the brain, that can affect neurons.

Normally, ammonia is cleared away quickly by the liver and disposed of in urine. However, the effects of liver, kidney disease or massive injury, producing excessive amounts of ammonia could stop this process happening.

The build-up of ammonia could damage brain cells.

Arginine – an amino acid – neutralises ammonia and is therefore useful for people with some neurodegenerative disorders.

There is less arginine in fish than meat. Nevertheless, fish is still a good source of arginine.

Gentle exercise is also essential for Increasing circulation to the liver and kidneys. This will help the process of removal of ammonia from the blood stream. Further, exercise will help retain muscle mass which is easily lost in MS.

Fish and Alanine

Alanine is a non-essential amino acid which means that your body can synthesise it. Its use is not directly related to the brain but it is used in the synthesis of carnosine which is another amino acid.

Carnosine has antioxidant benefits and helps to neutralise free radicals and reduce oxidative stress. In this respect, it is very useful as reducing oxidative stress and neutralising free radicals is to be desired in any form of neurodegeneration.

Excessive amounts of beta-alanine can cause paraesthesia. This manifests itself in the form of a tingling of the skin that is generally felt in the face, neck and back of the hand. It is harmless but, given that alanine is a non-essential amino acid, there is no reason why it should be supplemented since the body can make what it requires.

Further, alanine and taurine compete for absorption in the muscles and while we are unlikely to be deficient in beta alanine, most people are deficient in taurine.

The building blocks of myelin sheath

When we think about MS we know that the symptoms occur because the myelin sheath which surrounds the nerve and helps nerve impulses move along, is damaged.

Myelin sheath can and does repair itself. We know this because in the relapsing and remitting form of MS, the symptoms of a relapse occur during damage to the myelin and when it repairs itself – although it may be incomplete - this means that the disease has gone into remission.

This may be true in some cases but I do not believe that all symptoms generally associated with MS in those diagnosed with the condition has necessarily anything to do with demyelination.

However, for these purposes ……

The brain contains about 25% of all the cholesterol which is in your body and most of this is incorporated into your myelin sheath.

The cholesterol which is circulating in your body that is attached to lipoproteins is not the cholesterol that is used in the brain.

Bodily cholesterol cannot get past the blood brain barrier. Therefore, all the cholesterol forming nerve tissue is manufactured in the brain. Extra cholesterol is transported out of the brain.

Lipophilic statins cross the blood brain barrier more readily than hydrophilic ones. Although all stains can lead to central nervous system disorders

- Atorvastatin
- Lovastatin
- Simvastatin

as lipophilic statins tend to create more problems than the hydrophilic ones.

Common hydrophilic statins are:

- Pravastatin
- fluvastatin
- rosuvastatin

The use of statins has to be weighed up carefully in the light of the fact that impaired myelin synthesis may be the result of taking them.

Two main amino acids which are used in the synthesis of myelin sheath are:

- serine
- histidine

Histidine is important in the maintenance of myelin sheath. Histidine also boosts the action of suppressor T cells which are also known as Regulatory T cells. These cells help prevent autoimmune disease.

Histidine is found in most animal and vegetable proteins but are particularly high in:

- wheat germ
- poultry
- cheese
- pork

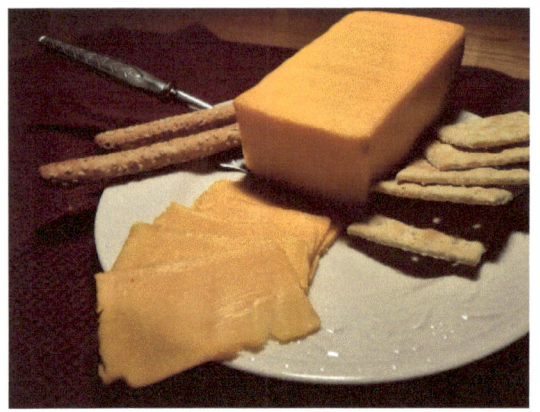

Cheese is a good source of histidine

As histidine is an essential amino acid, it must be taken in through food as it cannot be synthesised from other substances in the body.

Serine is a non-essential amino acid. This means that it can be produced in the human body but you will need the vitamin B complex, including folic acid, to do so.

Myelin sheath also needs serine as part of its composition. Without serine the sheaths would fray and become inefficient at delivering messages. Further, serine is part of all the proteins which form the brain.

If serine is so important which foods can it be found in?

Serine is synthesised from glycine which is the smallest amino acid that there is. Fish, meat, beans, milk and cheese, are the best dietary sources of glycine.

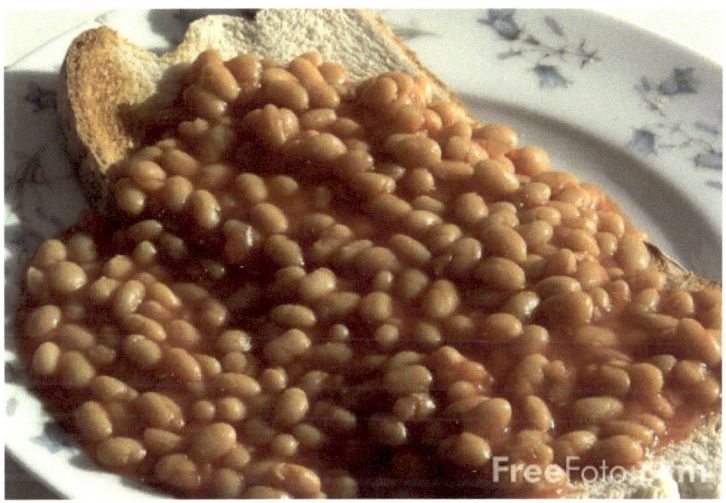

Beans are a good source of glycine

Vitamin C promotes re-myelination

Studies[12] have shown that vitamin C is essential in myelin formation. You will recall that oligodendrocytes make myelin sheath but, in order to do so, the immature oligodendrocytes must differentiate into mature oligodendrocytes. They cannot do this without sufficient vitamin C.

Vitamin C is found in fresh fruit and vegetables but it is very easily destroyed during cooking and storage so it is quite possible that insufficient vitamin C is taken in for the body's needs.

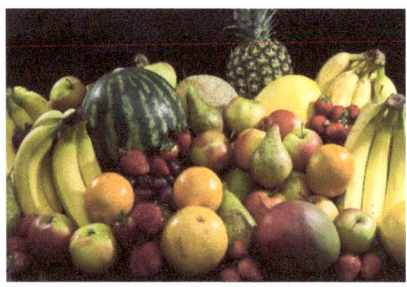

Fresh fruit and vegetables are a great source of vitamin C

---

[12] https://www.ncbi.nlm.nih.gov/pubmed/29423921

Cigarette smokers can use up a whole day's recommended daily allowance of vitamin C in a couple of cigarettes.

Alpha-lipoic acid is a fat AND water soluble powerful antioxidant. It has been found to reduce nerve damage symptoms such as numbness and pain. It is also involved in **nerve regeneration.**

Most studies[13] were conducted on people with diabetic neuropathy but ALA is also used by some medics for post herpetic neuralgia taken along with the vitamin B complex - which includes some vitamins B6 and B12 and folic acid – because of its nerve regenerating properties.

In a November 2016 article in Neurology Reviews, it was found that a daily oral intake of 1,200mg of lipoic acid significantly reduces the

---

[13] https://www.ncbi.nlm.nih.gov/pubmed/25381809

rate of whole brain atrophy among patients with secondary progressive MS.

It also helps to inhibit inappropriate microglial activation. Further, it was found to be safe and well tolerated.

ALA is also able to lower C-reactive protein that indicates chronic inflammation.

In animal models of MS, lipoic acid has been found to reduce inflammation and degeneration of the optic nerve and spinal cord.

Although there is no established daily dose, it is recommended that 600mg – 1,800mg is taken daily for three weeks for MS associated neuropathy.

ALA is found in very small amounts in many foods but the best sources of ALA are organ meats like liver, kidney and heart and red meat.

The practice of removing red meat from the diet, in MS, is not recommended because of the benefits of eating good sources of ALA.

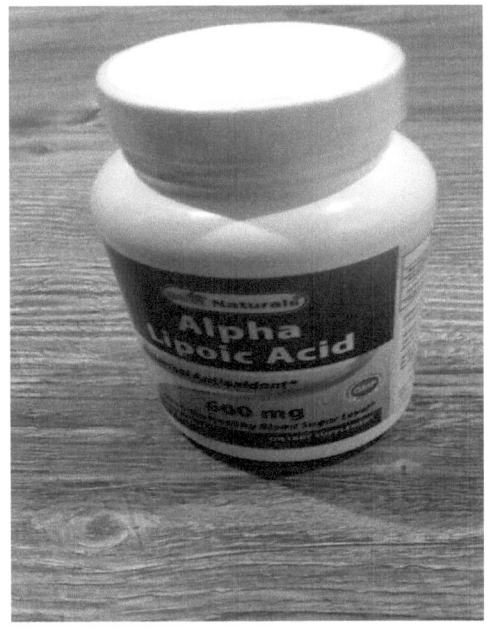

Vitamin B Complex

This complex consists of 8 vitamins: B1, B2, B3, B5, B6, B7, B9 and B12. They are water soluble vitamins. Some of these will be looked at individually below.

The effect of the B vitamins on neurological health is wide ranging. Some of this complex's functions impact on

- The maintenance of the myelin sheath which is a fatty sheath which surrounds nerve cells. Without this fatty coating, nerve signalling is impaired and affects motor function, cognition and mood.
- The Methylation Cycle
- The production and function of neurotransmitters

Vitamin B1 (Thiamine) – Thiamine was first discovered in 1926. It works synergistically with B2 and B6. It is easily destroyed by cooking, caffeine, food processing, alcohol and some drugs. Some studies have shown that lack of thiamine results in

- Poor or absent nerve impulses as it plays an essential role in nerve impulses
- Thiamine ensures that the brain and nerves have enough glucose for their requirements
- Studies have shown that thiamine deficiency has been shown to reduce the diameter of myelinic fibres as well as *increase cell death in the brain.*

Thiamine is so important that it is going to have a whole chapter to itself.

Good Sources of Thiamine

- Wholemeal grain
- Liver
- Eggs
- Pork
- Fish
- Nuts
- Green vegetables

- Fortified nutritional yeast is excellent.

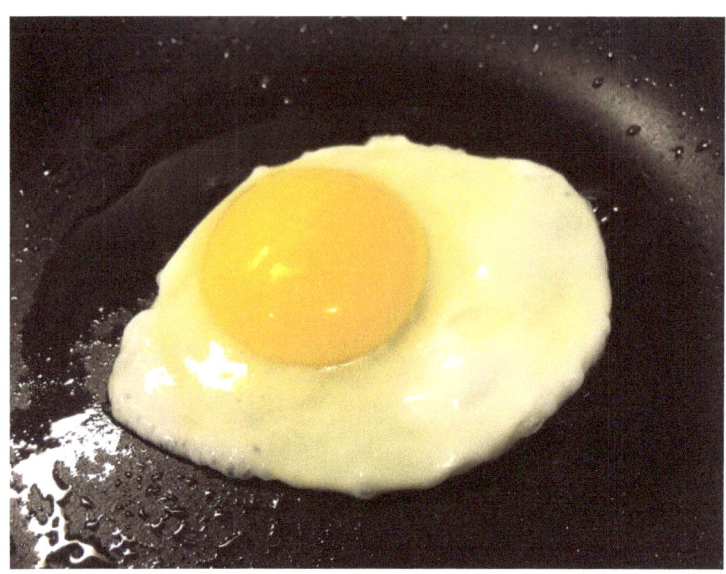

eggs are a great source of thiamine

Vitamin B3 (Niacin) – Niacin is necessary to maintain a healthy circulation to the brain. This helps maintain concentration and focus.

It is also a potent antioxidant and scavenges the free radicals which can set off neuro-inflammation.

I have already mentioned that microglia are cells in the brain which mop up inflammation and diseased cells.

An excess of microglia appears to be the 'wind fanning the flames' in the progression of neurodegeneration.

An adequate intake of niacin can therefore reduce the potential for inflammation in the first place and avoid rapid progression of neurodegeneration.

Interestingly, studies have also shown that quercetin and resveratrol reduced neuronal cell death instigated by microglial activation suggesting that they are potent anti-inflammatory compounds. We shall look at quercetin in more detail, later.

Resveratrol is found in red wine and grapes. The latter is the preferred form for taking in resveratrol since alcohol is toxic to the brain.

.

How niacin deficiency has the potential to lead to brain cell death.

Niacin is a forerunner to two coenzymes. Coenzymes are just non protein substances which are essential for enzymes to function.

These coenzymes are abbreviated to NAD and NADP.

NAD is needed to break down large substances into smaller ones. In this case it breaks down fats, carbohydrates and proteins into much smaller units.

NAD is also used to repair DNA and is involved in cell signalling.

NAD can convert to NADH and by a number of processes transfers food from diet into energy. If it is not required, it is stored as ATP.

ATP fuels the mitochondria which are the powerhouses in each cell.

The mitochondria produce the energy with which we need to survive.

If there isn't enough NADH then ATP will become depleted. Neuronal cell death is a potential outcome of this.

Vitamin B6 (Pyrioxidine)

Pyrioxidine helps make neurotransmitters and the protein, haemoglobin, which helps transport oxygen around the blood.

B6 is probably better known for maintaining normal levels of homocysteine which is an amino acid in the blood.

High levels of homocysteine are associated with cardiovascular disease.

In spite of this I have never known patients to be informed that it is homocysteine which is a contributory factor for heart disease rather than cholesterol.

This is not surprising given that a month's supply of vitamin B complex can be bought for as little as £2-£3 pounds off the supermarket shelf and cannot make profits for pharmaceutical companies in the way that statins can.

Vitamin B9 (Folic Acid) – studies undertaken at the University of Wisconsin, Madison on rats, suggests that folic acid may help promote healing in injured brains and spinal cord.

Vitamin B12 (Cobalamin) – this vitamin is essential for the development and function of brain and nerve cells. It helps promote the synthesis of lecithin which is a major component of the myelin sheath lipids.

There are only animal sources of Vitamin B12 and even then, this vitamin can only be separated from its food source in an acidic environment.

However, some nutritional yeasts are fortified with vitamin B12 and can be a useful addition to the diet since it can be sprinkled over food or stirred into soups and stews once they are cooked. Extended cooking can destroy some of the B vitamins.

Stomach acidity tends to reduce in older age and further many elderly individuals take antacids both of which impact on how well vitamin B12 can be absorbed.

Taking a little apple cider vinegar can help where there is loss of acidity and where reflux is a problem.

Further problems arise when there is loss of appetite often associated with illness and old age.

Studies have shown **marked increases in T regulatory cells** after vitamin B12 supplementation.

It is this increase in T regulatory cells which has been shown to slow down the rate of progression of neurodegenerative disease.

Vitamin B complex and the perils of smoking.

The vitamin B complex is easily destroyed by smoking which especially impacts vitamin B12.

Strangely enough studies have found that large doses of vitamin C also destroy vitamin B12.

The vitamin B complex is better taken first thing in the morning when vitamin C rich meals are less likely to be taken.

Further, B complex produces energy – something which you do not need a great deal of when you are trying to sleep. However, thiamine, vitamin B1, has been shown to aid sleep and works in the first day that it is taken. However, note that thiamine, like vitamin D, needs sufficient magnesium for its activation.

Magnesium is such a wonderful nutrient which is involved in hundreds of processes.

Sources of Vitamin B complex in food

As stated vitamin B12 is only found in animal sources – meat, fish, dairy and eggs. Vegetarians and vegans are therefore especially at risk of vitamin B12 deficiency.

Other forms of this B complex are generally found in meat, eggs, dairy and wholemeal foods such as bread, oats, and wheat germ. It is often added to breakfast cereals.

It is possible to be deficient in this complex given that it is so easily destroyed through a number of avenues.

Anyone with a neurodegenerative disorder should automatically have their B12 levels tested.

Given the importance of vitamin B complex in brain health, I would always recommend taking it in tablet form in addition to obtaining it from food although this complex is often added to cereals. It can be destroyed by cooking and is water soluble and is likely to leach out of foods when cooking. Needs for many nutrients rise when an individual is unwell but often appetite fails.

It can be found in supermarkets and is inexpensive.

Multiple sclerosis and the virus connection.

It has long been thought that there may be a virus, as yet undiscovered, that initiates multiple sclerosis. This is a plausible theory. Viruses are nasty things in spite of their miniscule size. They do not respond to antibiotics and so our defence is the ability of our immune system to detect and destroy these invaders.

Viruses are crafty. They hide inside our cells so that our immune system does not always know that they are there. Viruses hide around nerves because the immune system is less likely to attack and destroy them there. The immune system. If it does detect them, keeps them in check but doesn't go in for all-out war. To do so would damage vulnerable nervous tissue beyond repair.

The chicken pox virus is a case in point. It hides along nerves and remains hidden from childhood until older age. At this point the immune system is not functioning as well as it did in the younger body. The chicken pox virus emerges but now it is called shingles. The blistering and pain of shingles follows the nerve that the virus has hidden in for decades.

We can see how a virus can remain hidden in brain tissue, causing damage to the myelin sheath. The immune system cells cannot go for all-out war against the virus in the brain as it would destroy the host so the relapsing-remitting pattern of virus against immune system is in a double bind although, at some point, one will begin to win the battle.

Sometimes, MS appears to go away completely and sometimes it turns into a more progressive form with few, if any, relapses.

An insufficient amount of an amino acid, called lysine can lead to viral infections taking hold. It inhibits the ability of the virus to replicate.

Lysine is an essential amino acid and is found predominantly in animal protein such as:

- Beef
- Tuna
- Cheese
- Lamb
- poultry

Finally, we should not forget that taurine has many antimicrobial properties as has vitamin D. Both are to be found abundantly in the brain when there has been sufficient intake of these nutrients.

Thiamine

Thiamine is not a vitamin that takes precedence in most people's conversations when they are talking about vitamins. Most people know what vitamin D and C do, but ask them about thiamine and most people will shake their heads looking puzzled.

The importance of thiamine in the pathogenesis of many neurodegenerative disorders should not be overlooked. There is a world-wide deficiency of thiamine which is not recognised due to the mentality that developed countries like ours cannot possibly have a widespread deficiency disease.

We do not recognise it but, during the war years and immediate post war years, thiamine deficiency would be recognised by health care professionals quite easily.

Thiamine is a cofactor with enzymes that are connected with the mitochondrial function of all cells in the body.

The mitochondria are the power houses of each cell; tiny little organelles which generate most of the chemical energy needed to power the cell's biochemical reactions.

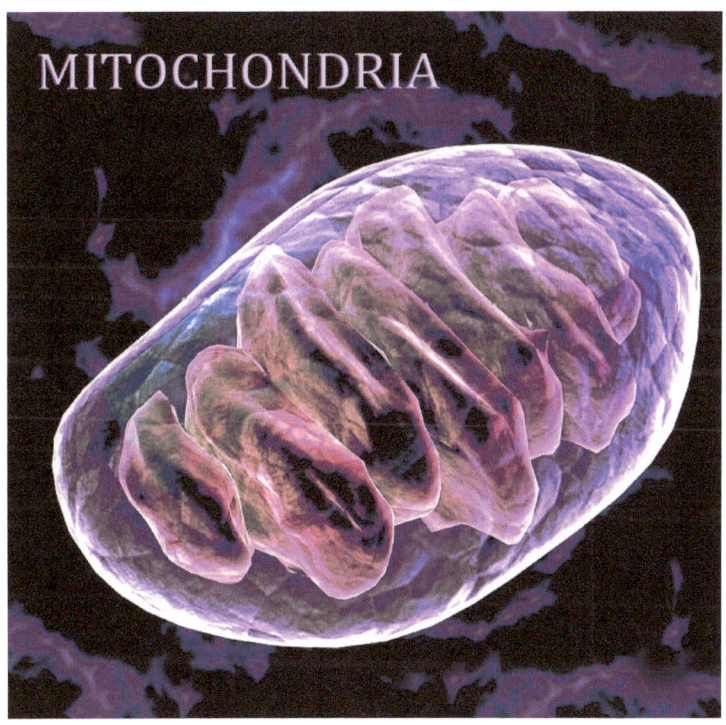

Mitochondria, powerhouses of the cell

The chemical energy is then stored in a tiny molecule known as adenosine triphosphate (ATP).

The fact that thiamine is needed in every cell of the body also means that when it isn't available, diverse and apparently unrelated signs and symptoms can occur.

Thiamine deficiency particularly impacts the nervous system in a condition called dry beriberi, the cardiovascular system – known as wet beriberi - and there is a form called gastrointestinal beriberi.

Symptoms of dry beriberi are diverse and encompass every symptom found in common neurodegenerative disorders including

  Multiple sclerosis

Motor neuron disease

Alzheimer's disease

Parkinson's disease

Vascular dementia

and many more

Thiamine deficiency can cause unsteady gait, nystagmus, tingling, burning sensation, aphasia, dysphasia, slurred speech, problems with word finding, bowel and bladder problems, weakness, fatigue, depression, anxiety, stabbing pain, joint pain, tremor and muscle weakness. Indeed, any symptom that you might associate with a diagnosis of multiple sclerosis.

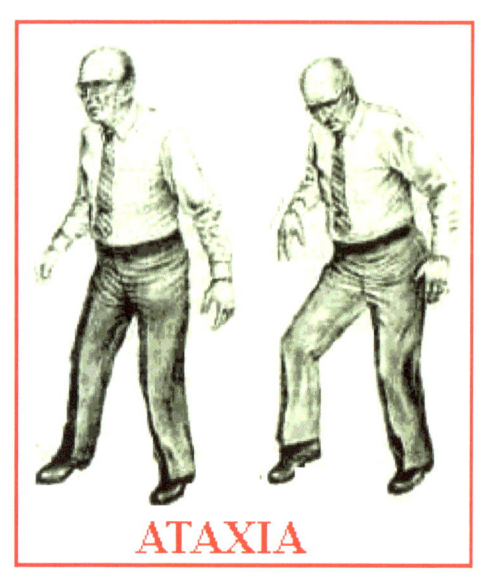
ATAXIA

Can thiamine deficiency explain remitting relapsing MS or primary progressive or secondary progressive? Well yes, it can.

Let us take the remitting relapse MS. A person who is borderline in thiamine may at times drop below the amount needed for health. The familiar symptoms, associated with MS will manifest themselves but if a diet rich in thiamine is eaten then the symptoms will improve within hours and the 'relapse' will have remitted.

This is really nothing to do with autoimmunity. It is purely the result of an easily correctable nutritional deficiency.

If the patient is thiamine insufficient (or deficient in the activating magnesium – or both) and this is not corrected, then they may permanently find themselves below the level of thiamine needed for good health. They will manifest symptoms of dry beriberi which are exactly as described in those with MS.

A primary progressive diagnosis may be due to permanently poor eating habits which may never resolve and, as such, the condition will continue to deteriorate without any chance to resolve. Make no mistake thiamine deficiency impacts the quality of life but can also result in death.

For all that researchers have spent decades trying to unravel the mystery of MS, it is still not known whether it is a genuine autoimmune disease or a manifestation of something else. We often hear, 'We don't really know what causes MS but we believe it is this, this and this. However, thinking is an assumption. It may be a good one but it may lead us away from something that is looking at us directly in the face.

Reduced thiamine can result in plaques and fibrotic tissue, among others which, on an MRI scan, may point to a diagnosis of MS but then this should lead us to consider the possibility of a nutritional deficiency.

Why do we not consider beriberi? Why do we not recognise that the signs and symptoms of MS may be dry beriberi which, with treatment, can for the most part be reversed in days although full effect in severe cases may take up to 6 months.

Could one of the reasons be that, treating a deficiency disease with a supplement is not profitable for drug's companies. I don't know. I do know though that there are research papers galore that cite MS as being a manifestation of beriberi but nothing, of value, appears to develop from that.

While, I understand that people with some cognitive disorder are tested for vitamin B12 deficiency, they are not tested for thiamine deficiency. This is puzzling given the devastating impact that dry beriberi can have if it is not treated in time.

Our diet lacks thiamine now. It is added to white flour but bioavailability may be an issue. The foods we used to eat in the 1950's to address any deficiency which may occur are no longer eaten regularly. For example, lightly cooked liver is an excellent source of thiamine and was served at least once a week in the 1950's. Malted milk and malt spread were drunk or eaten on a daily basis in most households. Both are rich sources of thiamine. Peanut butter was the spread that appeared on everyone's table often proving more popular than jam. Nuts are an incredibly rich source of thiamine as is wholemeal bread and grains.

Yogurt and milk are excellent sources of thiamine too but dairy milk is not as popular and children do not receive a third of a pint of milk at school which used to be the usual practice in the 1950's until the 1970's when the prime minister, Margaret Thatcher, became known as Margaret Thatcher, the milk snatcher when she removed the free milk provided at school/

Thiaminase is an enzyme which breaks down thiamine so that it cannot be used. Thiaminase is found in tea, coffee, raw fish (think shellfish and sushi) high carbohydrate diets and alcohol. These are all habits that have become popular and almost certainly destroy most, if not all, of the thiamine in an already thiamine poor diet.

The fatigue and depression that ensue are put down to many things - unhealthy family relationships, work related stress, MS - among others. The reality is that thiamine deficiency – and the psychiatric symptoms such as irritability, anger and depression that are characteristic of

It can actually be the driving force of unhealthy family relationships or be responsible for such fatigue that work no longer holds any challenge or enjoyment.

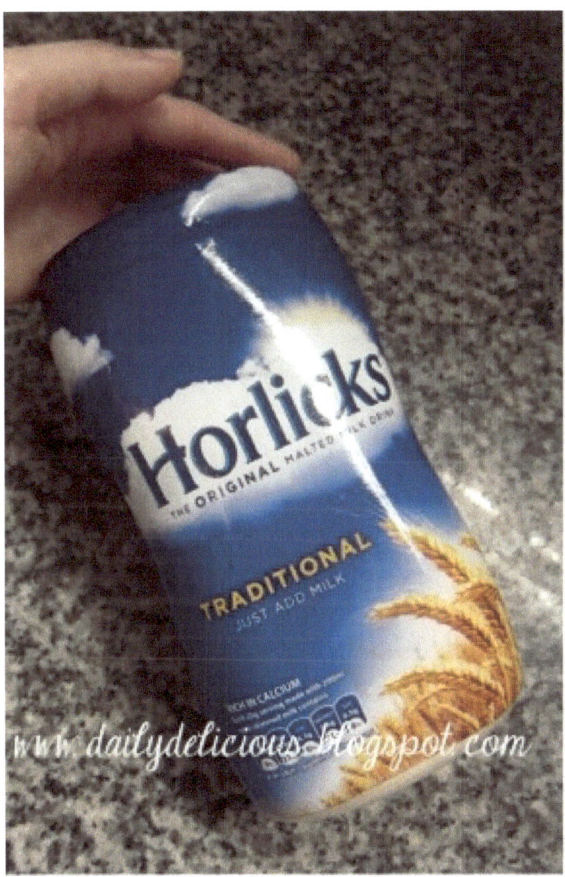

Malted milk – full of thiamine and other B vitamins

The recommended dietary allowance for thiamine is 1.2mg and 1.4mg for pregnant women. However, this appears to be far too low. Many people do not begin to get relief until much higher, therapeutic doses are given. Indeed, for cognitive decline the recommended dose is 500mg three times daily with those suffering from Parkinson's disease treated with up to 4g (4.000mg) daily.

Those diagnosed with MS could try 300mg daily in divided doses if this is better but at least 300mg should be taken daily in order to activate the thiamine.

Once a therapeutic dose is reached then the results are quite dramatic. People begin to sleep soundly through the night, they no longer need an afternoon nap, they suddenly get up out of their chairs, after sitting doing nothing for weeks, and begin to do the housework or the cooking. They become more sociable, they are steadier on their feet, they remember where they put their glasses down. There aches and pains, muscle spasms, seizures, bowel problems begin to resolve.

This was no autoimmune disease or part of the ageing process at all, it is the result of a largely unrecognised vitamin deficiency.

We should not leave this chapter on MS and the fact that it may be a manifestation of beri beri without looking at the gastrointestinal form of beri beri. This is the new kid on the block; the most recently recognised of thiamine deficiency with its countless faces leading to some saying. ' are most conditions just a manifestation of thiamine deficiency? Well, there's a thought!

Gastrointestinal beriberi manifests itself in gastroparesis type symptoms which include:

- intractable constipation
- bloating
- upper and lower abdominal discomfort
- delayed transit
- pain
- indigestion (due to delayed gastric emptying and poor tone of oesophageal

valve which allows stomach contents back up into the oesophagus – lax sphincter valves can occur due to poor stomach acidity; another symptom of thiamine deficiency)

As thiamine deficiency becomes more profound, those diagnosed with MS tend to end up at the Bladder and Bowel clinics. In fact, it is thought that the more advanced cases of MS are to be found there although this may well result from a longer slide into beriberi through prolonged B1 deficiency (and/or magnesium deficiency)

Thiamine cannot harm and so it is worth trying. It may take a few weeks to begin to correct a deficiency involving the gastrointestinal tract whereas the impact on mental health and sleep may occur immediately.

2g of vitamin C during this time may also help although vitamin C should always be taken at the opposite end of the day to the B complex.

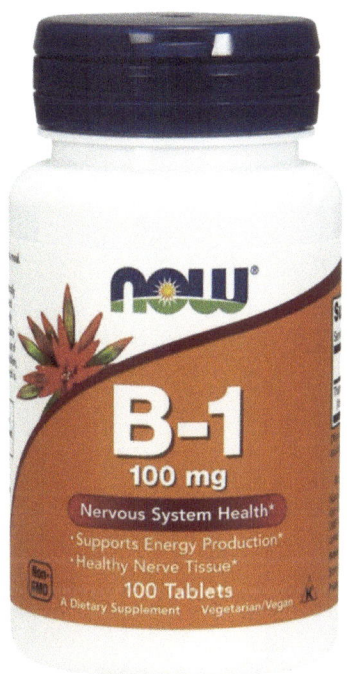

Thiamine – a cure for all ills?

Thiamine, Sources, Functions and other Miscellany

Best food sources:

Dried Brewer's yeast

Fortified nutritional yeast flakes

Yeast extract

Brown rice

Wheat germ

Nuts

Liver

Wholemeal bread

Please note that as thiamine is susceptible to heat. It is destroyed easily. As such, although it may say that any item contains a certain amount to thiamine, that does not mean that

such an amount is being ingested. Even then, the amount absorbed in the gut will be less than that.

The thiamine added to food is not necessarily bioavailable and there are no safeguards to compel a bioavailable form of thiamine.

In addition, the amount of carbohydrate that is normally present with thiamine tends to use it up rapidly leaving none for other functions in the body.

Lightly cooked pork liver is a good source as is yeast extract but the only safe way to get adequate amounts in a neurodegenerative disorder is to supplement in high with magnesium. Thiamine has no known side effects at high doses and has not been found to interact with any medications.

Deficiency symptoms

MS and other neurodegenerative disorders like Parkinson's Disease, Alzheimer's Disease and Motor Neuron Disease
Tingling and burning in the feet, stabbing pains
Fatigue
Tender calves and overall fibromyalgia type pain
Poor concentration, brain fog
Impaired memory
Muscle weakness
Loss of appetite
Depression and irritability and anxiety
Digestive upsets including constipation, bloating, abdominal discomfort in general, indigestion, heartburn
Indigestion (thiamine is required to keep the stomach acidic and close the valve at the top of the stomach

nausea
Insomnia and poor sleep patterns

Deficiency caused by:

alcohol
High carbohydrate diets
Black coffee and tea
Poor diet, malnutrition and subnutrition
Pregnancy
Breast feeding
Fever
Gastrointestinal Surgery and surgery in general
Antacid drugs like the proton pump inhibitors
Physical stress
Mental stress
Infection and trauma

Therapeutic Uses

Beri beri
Improved ability to focus and concentrate – similar effect to Modafinil
Repels insects
Useful in indigestion
Improving cardiac function
Required in cases of heavy drinking and alcoholism
Nerve injury – lumbago, trigeminal neuralgia, sciatica, Bell's Palsy, optic neuritis
Insomnia

Beri-beri is a little known condition now. During the second World War it was part of the curriculum of school age children since it was rife. It still is rife but knowledge about it has largely been neglected in more recent times. It was, in the 1950's part of the junior school curriculum and everyone was encouraged to eat more offal, yeast extract, Ovaltine, malt, Brewer's yeast and similar in order to obtain the amounts that they needed.

Most of these foods have now fallen out of fashion. Thiamine manifests itself in countless ways but is not recognised as such. Those with heart failure will be given pharmaceutical medicines but tests for thiamine deficiency are never given.

Those with neurodegenerative disorders will be given tests for vitamin B12 deficiency but never for thiamine deficiency which helps maintain the acidic environment that vitamin B12 requires for its absorption.

Thiamine simply is a co-enzyme converting glucose into energy in muscles and nerves.

Trying to live without thiamine is like trying to get a car to move when it has run out of petrol.

In the early deficiency stages everything will be hard work. If the deficiency is not corrected then speech will falter, ability to recall information will become more apparent, even getting out of a chair will be a hurdle. When handling things they will appear 'heavy.'

It is far easier to correct this in the earlier stages when repair to damaged nerves and muscles may not take as long to correct. Severely damaged nerves can take up to a year to repair but once thiamine is taken to start addressing the damage caused by the deficiency the subtle improvements can be seen almost immediately and build up day by day.

I have known people in their mid-70's who were unable to walk down steps without holding onto a rail, take thiamine for a week and then skip down the middle of the steps without the need to hold onto anything. Until you have experienced this for yourself it is difficult to understand the miraculous properties of thiamine.

Just remember that thiamine needs to be stored in a cool dark place. Sunlight destroys thiamine and this is why yeast extract is always sold in a dark glass jar and yeast flakes are kept in foil insulated packing normally.

Vitamin C Deficiency and MS

The problems with some vitamins is that they get a certain reputation so for example, we take vitamin D for our bones and Vitamin C, so the story goes, is useful to shorten a common cold. We can be quite blinkered about some nutrients and forget that they will be involved in numerous processes inside the body which are just as, if not more important, than the popular knowledge we have been fed with.

Before we start looking at vitamin C and some of the many other functions it has it needs to be stated that vitamin C is not citric acid. Vitamin C is ascorbic acid and is normally found as sodium ascorbate in supplements.

Vitamin C is a vital antioxidant in the brain which is necessary where injury and infection may have increased microglia activation.

It is certainly needed for myelin formation. Targeted deletion of a sodium-vitamin C co-transporter has been found to cause cerebral haemorrhage in diverse areas of the brain.

We do know that vitamin C deficiency is manifested in many mental health disorders such as depression and anxiety, general malaise and more complex conditions like schizophrenia and other psychoses. Could it be that the general fatigue that those with MS complain about is due to a vitamin C deficiency?

Vitamin C is needed for the synthesis of an amino acid known as carnitine. One of carnitine's functions is to oxidise stored fat and use it to create energy. The impact that one gram of vitamin C can make is noticeable in terms of lightened mood and increased energy.

Vitamin C has the ability to pull water back into the gut thus making the passage of stool much easier. The phenomenon of 'bowel tolerance' when deciding how much vitamin C is appropriate for your use is well known.

It is far better to take something like vitamin C than a number of the bowel aiding medications that are on offer such as the indigestible sugars, the medications that you mix with water than contain lots of minerals to aid function but, all too often, overdo it, so that you daren't go out anywhere. Then there are the stimulants which can give you pain as they force the contents to expel themselves along the gut.

The gastrointestinal system is such a delicate system which deserves far better than we give it.

When the transport of vitamin C is disrupted studies have shown that it contributes to brain damage in premature infants.

Vitamin C deficiency is also known to impair memory and is known to bring about pathological problems when there has been exposure to neurotoxins like aluminium.

In fact, concentrations of vitamin C are found to be at their highest in the central nervous system which appears to be a little known fact.

Really, if the brain depends on vitamin C so much then any neurological manifestation is possible – poor balance, gastro-intestinal issues, poor memory recall, slurring of speech and so on.

Constipation is a symptom of MS, often due to slower transit which means that most of the fluid is absorbed back into the system. Vitamin C has the opposite effect and pulls fluid back into the gut.

A Japanese study also evidences how sufficient vitamin C is needed for physical performance including balance. This study involved 655 subjects living in Tokyo, Japan. They did not take supplements.

Those with a higher vitamin C concentration had better handgrip strength. They could stand up for longer periods on one legs with their eyes open and they could walk faster.

The conclusion drawn was that in elderly women the higher the concentration of plasma vitamin C the better the muscle strength and overall physical performance.

Overall physical performance and physical activity is linked with future disability, morbidity and death[14]

Since vitamin C is needed for remyelination then insufficient vitamin C for someone's needs is able to induce the symptoms that that are characteristic of MS.

Some of the medications dished out today are often inappropriately given. For example, people with swollen ankles are given diuretics which helps remove the fluid. However, it is quite common to find that this fluid retention responds well to vitamin B1 (with magnesium). If diuretics are continued they unfortunately also flush out the water soluble vitamin C.

Vitamin C has a little known therapeutic action on people with allergies who often find they retain fluid as part of their condition.

---

[14] Bartali B et al Age and disability affect dietary intake J Nutr, 2003 vol 133 page 2868- 2873

Vitamin C reduces the synthesis of histamine which is responsible for the leakiness of the vessels which results in fluid retention. It works slightly differently from antihistamines which block the histamine receptors found on cells. Once these receptors are blocked, histamine cannot exert its effects on cells.

Although there does not appear to be a direct link between MS and allergies it should be borne in mind that inflammation and histamine are associated. Further, allergies can cause some of the symptoms associated with MS such as brain fog and fatigue.

In effect, we can explain all the well-established characteristics of MS on a vitamin C deficiency.

The Recommended Daily Intake (RDI) of vitamin C is 75mg for adult women and 90mg for adult males. This appears wholly adequate and it appears that this RDI was set at these levels in order to avoid scurvy but did not really contribute to the glowing health that high serum vitamin C levels are capable of producing.

Moreover, our lifestyles have changed since these RDI's were set. Just as an example, seed oils are inflammatory in nature whereas the saturated animal fats are not. As we have replaced animal fats (lard butter and dripping) with seed oils, our need for vitamin c, (just in this respect) has increased. We tend to buy more store bought food instead of growing it ourselves and picking it as needed. Vitamin C is easily lost in storage and so the fruit and vegetables in supermarkets may contain little, if any, vitamin C.

I am sure that you can think of many more examples which have had a negative impact on our daily intake of vitamin C.

Any tissue injury requires huge amounts of vitamin C in order for it to heal. This includes such events as tooth extractions, fractures, burns, scalds and major trauma.

At times such as these, vitamin C intake needs to be increased dramatically so that there is not only enough for tissue healing but to keep the other tissues and organs functioning optimally on a daily basis.

Table 2: Vitamin C Content of Selected Foods [12]

Food	Milligrams (mg) per serving	Percent (%) DV*
Red pepper, sweet, raw, ½ cup	95	106
Orange juice, ¾ cup	93	103
Orange, 1 medium	70	78
Grapefruit juice, ¾ cup	70	78
Kiwifruit, 1 medium	64	71
Green pepper, sweet, raw, ½ cup	60	67
Broccoli, cooked, ½ cup	51	57
Strawberries, fresh, sliced, ½ cup	49	54
Brussels sprouts, cooked, ½ cup	48	53
Grapefruit, ½ medium	39	43
Broccoli, raw, ½ cup	39	43
Tomato juice, ¾ cup	33	37
Cantaloupe, ½ cup	29	32
Cabbage, cooked, ½ cup	28	31
Cauliflower, raw, ½ cup	26	29
Potato, baked, 1 medium	17	19
Tomato, raw, 1 medium	17	19
Spinach, cooked, ½ cup	9	10
Green peas, frozen, cooked, ½ cup	8	9

https://ods.od.nih.gov/factsheets/VitaminC-HealthProfessional/#h3

Pulling it all together

There isn't any one test that can definitely diagnose MS. A diagnosis is made on:

- finding evidence of damage in at least two separate areas of the central nervous system which includes the spinal cord, brain and optic nerves.

AND

- find evidence that the areas of damage occurred at two different points of time at least.

AND

- rule out other possible diagnoses

While this criterion may lead to a diagnosis of MS, it doesn't actually tell us what is causing these areas of damage. It is possible that the areas of damage – lesions - in MS may be caused by different things but manifest itself similarly in various individuals.

We have already seen that excessive ammonia can damage neurons as can excessive salt in cells. Here we have different ways that damage to nerve cells can occur but both will result in the classic MS lesions.

Regardless of the underlying cause, it is prudent to keep vitamin D levels up due to its regulatory effect on the immune system and its anti-microbial effects. It responds to a faulty dysregulated immune system and any infective agent.

Paying attention to thiamine levels is of paramount importance because of the increasing belief now that most neurodegenerative disorders are just a manifestation of a thiamine deficiency where perceived differences may just be a manifestation of genetic diversity. It does cover all the bases and supplementing with thiamine has shown time and time again to reverse the symptoms belonging to another diagnosed condition.

A low salt/no salt diet is always to be sought since there is enough salt in the diet anyway. Adding high blood pressure to MS – which may both have its roots in excessive salt - is just adding insult to injury. Taurine – with its diuretic effect - can deal with this type of difficulty, allowing astrocytes to be able to function correctly and exert their neuroprotective effects.

Once myelin sheath is damaged we need to provide the right building blocks to help rebuild it and the role of vitamin C has also been discussed, among others, in this book. However, vitamin C has a wider role than just building myelin sheath; it's importance needs to be borne in mind.

There is generally an interplay of genetic and environmental factors underpinning multiple sclerosis and taking any one of the factors out of the equation may positively change the course of the disease.

Not everything written in the genes will come to fruition. Genes can be turned on and off – that is regulated by something such as vitamin D. This is an example of the interaction of genetic and environmental factors and how environmental factors such as nutrition can turn the switch off that makes someone vulnerable to a particular condition.

Your body is designed to heal itself but in order to do so it requires the correct building blocks to do so. Taking vital food groups out, which occurred in the Swank diet, can remove vital nutrients from the diet which can not only progress MS but introduce other diseases of malnutrition as well.

Most people, with any illness, know instinctively what makes them feel better and what makes them feel worse. MS is no different.

In 1996 when I was diagnosed with relapsing-remitting MS, I started taking extra vitamin D as my diet was deficient. Knowing the value of the B complex vitamins, I added that to my supplements. I already had an aversion to salt and had refused to add it to any of my cooking for many years.

I have remained symptom free, from MS, ever since. That is, for over 35 years.

Thank you for purchasing this book.

Every time a book is purchased, a donation is made to one of the charities I am currently supporting. These can be found on the author's website.

See below.

Other Health Related Books by the Author

- The Reluctant Bowel
- A Weighty Issue
- Sleep, Perchance to Dream
- The Journey: EDS and chronic pain
- The MND diet: using nutrition to slow down the progress of neurodegeneration

- A Necessary Sorrow
- Treat infection Naturally
- Successful Aging
- Taking another Road: Pain: its causes and what can be done about it
- Osteoarthritis and Pain
- A Treatment Strategy for Migraine

These can be found here on the author's page

https://www.amazon.co.uk/-/e/B07BPQZ5CD

Lynne writes regular articles and protocols for various medical conditions which can be found on her website here:

https://www.buymeacoffee.com/lynnedmnobl

Please help support this valuable work and please pass the link onto friends and family,